SAQs for the MRCPsych Part II

Dr Michael I Levi
MB, BS(Lond.), MRCPsych Part I
Registrar to the Professorial Unit of Psychiatry,
The London Hospital, Whitechapel,
London, UK

with a Foreword by
Professor S I Cohen
Professor of Psychiatry, The London Hospital Medical College,
University of London, UK

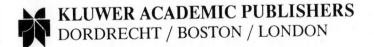

KLUWER ACADEMIC PUBLISHERS
DORDRECHT / BOSTON / LONDON

Distributors

for the United States and Canada: Kluwer Academic Publishers, PO Box 358, Accord
Station, Hingham, MA 02018-0358, USA
for all other countries: Kluwer Academic Publishers Group, Distribution Center, PO Box
322, 3300 AH Dordrecht, The Netherlands

British Library Cataloguing in Publication Data

Levi, Michael I, *1960*–
    SAQs for the MRCPsych part II.
    1. Medicine. Psychiatry – Questions &
    answers
    I. Title
    616.89'0076

    ISBN 0-7462-0099-4

Copyright

Published in the United Kingdom by Kluwer Academic Publishers, PO Box 55,
Lancaster, UK.

Kluwer Academic Publishers BV incorporates the publishing programmes of D. Reidel,
Martinus Nijhoff, Dr W. Junk and MTP Press.

Printed in Great Britain by Butler and Tanner, Frome and London.

Contents

Foreword

There has always been argument as to whether clinical subjects can be examined through multiple choice questions (MCQs) or short answer questions (SAQs) and most agree that it is not easy to set such questions in a subject like psychiatry. It is often easier to set questions on what might be called the small print of psychiatry than on the important main issues, knowledge of which should indicate that a candidate has received a comprehensive training in psychiatry and in the related sciences, is now a competent clinician and is capable of proceeding to higher training. Despite this difficulty these types of questions seem to have come to stay and SAQs seem to me to be much more relevant than MCQs to a clinical subject like psychiatry. In this book Dr Levi presents a structured aid to candidates which should ensure that their technique in answering the questions on the day is adequate to the task. Although the book contains a great deal of factual information it is not intended as a brief summary of 'psychiatry for the membership' but it will be a great help to candidates in assuring that if they have been adequately trained and have read sufficiently widely they will not fail because of lack of examination techniques.

Samuel I Cohen
Professor of Psychiatry
The London Hospital Medical College

Introduction

As from May 1988, the membership examination for the MRCPsych has changed its format considerably. It has also changed its name to the MRCPsych Part II. For details of these changes, may I refer the reader to the introductory section of my second book[1].

A major change in the MRCPsych Part II is the inclusion of a short answer question (SAQ) paper, which did not occur in the membership examination. The candidate has to answer 20 compulsory questions in 90 minutes. Equal emphasis will be placed on basic sciences and clinical topics in psychiatry i.e. there will be the same number of questions under each of these headings; this may necessitate the use of integrated questions.

The purpose of writing this book is to give candidates for the MRCPsych Part II adequate practice at the types of SAQ they will encounter. The 200 SAQs in this book have been distributed equally between basic sciences and clinical topics i.e. in the same proportion as the candidate will find in the exam.

I have based my questions on two books of revision notes – one covering basic sciences[2], the other covering clinical topics[3]. These books are very useful for this part of the examination, since they provide lists of information in a form very similar to the short answer. Candidates will benefit most by attempting each SAQ in 4½ minutes, the allocated time in the MRCPsych Part II. They should then look up the answer to the question at the back of the book.

The subject matter and distribution of questions in this book is based on the sample SAQ paper issued by the Royal College of Psychiatrists.

References

1. Levi, M.I. (1988). *MCQs for the MRCPsych Part II* (Lancaster: Kluwer Academic Publishers)
2. Dinan, T.G. (1985). *Examination Notes on the Scientific Basis of Psychiatry* (Bristol: John Wright)
3. Bird, J. and Harrison, G. (1987). *Examination Notes in Psychiatry* (Bristol: John Wright)

Examination Technique

The most important principle in answering the SAQ is to keep the answer brief and to the point. The candidate must read each question carefully and answer only what is asked. The answer should be in a list of information or brief notes.

Remember, the examiner has a checklist of certain points he is looking for when marking each SAQ – and it is on this basis that he passes or fails the candidate. It is better to list 5 relevant points than to write a long-winded paragraph of generalisations. The latter might appear more impressive, but will score less than the former.

Quick thinking is also required in this part of the examination. Only 4½ minutes are allowed for each SAQ. The first 1½ minutes should be spent planning the answer; scribbling some notes or key words in rough might help the candidate to jog his memory. I advise candidates initially to go through all the questions that they feel they can answer readily. They should then go back and attempt the questions they are less sure about. This technique ensures that candidates maximise the amount of factual information imparted to the examiners.

Finally, don't panic! Everyone is in the same situation as you are, and you can only do your best. Don't try to be too clever when answering the SAQs – keep the answers relatively simple.

Acknowledgements

I wish to thank Professor S I Cohen for writing the Foreword to this book and for the privilege of working for him on the Professorial Unit of Psychiatry at the London Hospital.

I also wish to thank Dr M A Reveley and Dr D Roy for appointing me to the London Hospital Rotational Training Scheme in Psychiatry, involving Tower Hamlets, Redbridge and Newham Health Authorities.

I am also very grateful to Dr A Margo at Goodmayes Hospital for providing an intellectually stimulating environment for my first job on the rotation.

Thanks yet again to Dr J M Brewis of Kluwer Academic Publishers for giving me the opportunity of publishing my third book.

A special thank-you must go to Mr S Ogrodzinski of Duphar Laboratories Ltd, who helped me to secure the publication of my material.

Finally, thanks once again to my parents for their motivating influence.

Basic Sciences

1. List 3 examples of glycerophospholipids and 3 examples of sphingolipids.
    Briefly describe the function of each.

2. Write short notes on the evidence for and against the dopamine theory of schizophrenia.

3. List 4 criteria a substance should fulfil to be classified as a neurotransmitter.

4. Name 2 important pyrimidine bases and 2 important purine bases.
    List four processes they are involved in.

5. Write short notes on the evidence for the monoamine theory of depression.

6. List 3 characteristics each for the nicotinic and muscarinic responses to acetylcholine.

7. Name the final breakdown products resulting from the catabolism of serotonin, dopamine and noradrenaline.
    Name the enzymes involved in the catabolism of these catecholamines.

8. Name 12 neurotransmitters.

9. List 5 of the intermediate substances involved in the Embden–Meyerhof pathway.

10. Define the terms resting membrane potential and action potential.
    On which ions is each dependent?

11. List the types of waves seen in an electroencephalogram (EEG) together with their frequency ranges.
    Name the EEG characteristic typical of delirious states.

12. Define the terms IPSPs and EPSPs.
    What are the underlying ionic changes in each?

13. List the uses of the EEG in psychiatry.

14. List the 5 types of synaptic contact.

15. Write short notes on the EEG changes during non-REM sleep.

16. List the different groups of neuroleptics (major tranquillizers) with one example of a drug in each group.

17. List 5 distinct biochemical actions attributable to neuroleptics.
    Define the origin of the name largactil.

18. List the clinical indications for chlorpromazine.

19. Write short notes on the mechanism by which lithium is thought to produce its therapeutic effects.

20. List the long-term side-effects of lithium.

21. List the clinical indications for lithium.

22. List 10 major drugs which interact with monoamine oxidase inhibitors (MAOIs).

23. Define tardive dyskinesia.
    List 7 possible treatments.

24. Classify tricyclic antidepressants into two types of compound. Give the characteristic feature and 2 examples of each type of compound.

25. Name the diencephalic, metencephalic and mesencephalic structures.

26. Name the structures involved in the direct and consensual light reflexes.

27. Name the components, principal inputs and principal outputs of the basal ganglia.

28. Name the locations of noradrenergic neurones in the brain.
    List their projections.

29. List the 6 layers of the cerebral cortex.

30. Name the structures involved in the accommodation reflex.

31. Name the components, principal inputs and principal outputs of the limbic system.

32. Name the locations of dopaminergic neurones in the brain.
    List their projections.

33. List the positions and names of the nuclei in the hypothalamus.

34. List the clinical features of Addison's disease.

35. Write short notes on the hypothalamic – pituitary – thyroid axis.

36. List the clinical features of the menopause.

37. Name the principal stimulatory and inhibitory hypothalamic hormones.

38. List the clinical features of phaeochromocytoma.

39. Write short notes on the hypothalamic – pituitary – gonadal axis.

40. List 6 endocrine abnormalities in anorexia nervosa.

41. Write short notes on the principal types of genetic studies in psychiatry.

42. List the clinical features of homocystinuria.
    What is the enzyme deficiency, mode of inheritance and treatment of the condition?

43. List the clinical features of Hurler's syndrome.
    What are the differences between Hunter's syndrome and Hurler's syndrome?

44. List the clinical features of Klinefelter's syndrome.
Define the genotype.

45. List the clinical features of phenylketonuria.
What is the enzyme deficiency, mode of inheritance and
treatment of the condition?

46. List the clinical features of galactosaemia.
What is the enzyme deficiency and treatment of the condition?

47. List the clinical features of tuberous sclerosis.
What is the mode of inheritance?

48. List the clinical features of Turner's syndrome.
Define the genotype.

49. List 10 clinical features of the frontal lobe syndrome.

50. List the clinical features of Alzheimer's disease.
Describe the pathology of the condition.

51. Outline the clinical features of Wernicke's encephalopathy and
Korsakoff's psychosis.

52. List the clinical features of disseminated sclerosis.

53. List the clinical features of the parietal lobe syndrome.

54. List the clinical features of multi-infarct dementia.
Describe the pathology of the condition.

55. Write short notes on the aetiology, pathology, clinical features and prognosis of the punch-drunk syndrome.

56. Write short notes on the metabolic error, clinical features and mode of inheritance of acute intermittent porphyria.

57. Outline the principal differences between classical and operant conditioning.

58. List the names of 6 neo-freudians and 6 post-freudians.

59. Define Piaget's 4 stages in cognitive development.
List the characteristics of each stage.

60. List the characteristic features of Adler's school of individual psychology.

61. List the characteristic features of short-term and long-term memory.

62. Name 12 ego-defence mechanisms.

63. Define Freud's 5 stages of psychosexual development.
List the characteristics of each stage.

64. Describe briefly the 4 stages involved in the treatment of phobic disorders by systematic desensitization.

65. Define the following terms – extracampine visual hallucination, autoscopic hallucination, reflex hallucination and complex hallucination.

66. Write short notes on the 3 subgroups of disorders of the form of thought.

67. Define and contrast the terms delusion and overvalued idea.

68. Describe briefly the 5 forms in which obsession can occur.

69. Define the terms Gedankenlautwerden and écho de la pensée.

70. List the characteristic features of hallucinations and pseudohallucinations.

71. Define the terms primary delusion and secondary delusion.

72. Define the terms illusion de sosies and Fregoli's illusion.

73. Define the prevalence rates of generalized anxiety disorders, obsessional – compulsive disorders, affective disorders, schizophrenia and Alzheimer's disease.

74. List the characteristic features of parametric and non-parametric statistical tests.
    Which is preferable and why?

75. Define the terms reliability and validity.
    List 3 types of reliability and 2 types of validity.

76. Define the terms incidence and prevalence.
    How is each calculated?

77. Write short notes on the 3 types of epidemiological observational studies.

78. Define the terms type I error and type II error in hypothesis testing.
How do they inter-relate?

79. Define the statistical method known as analysis of variance (ANOVA).
What situations are one-way ANOVA and two-way ANOVA used in?

80. Define the terms target population, sample population, random sample and stratified random sample.

81. Name the 5 axes in the DSM III system of classification.

82. Name the 4 classes in Fould's hierarchical classification.
What did Foulds mean by the term hierarchy?

83. Define the terms categorical and non-categorical classification.

84. Define the term labelling theory.
What are its consequences?

85. Write short notes on the differences between the ICD-9 and DSM III systems of classification.

86. Write short notes on the findings of the US – UK Diagnostic Project (1972) and the International Pilot Study of Schizophrenia (1973) in relation to diagnostic criteria.

87.   Define the conditions bouffée délirante and délires chroniques.

88.   Write short notes on the BPRS and PSE standardized interviews.

89.   Define the 5 social classes in relation to occupation.
      Define the social causation and social drift hypotheses of
      schizophrenia.

90.   List the characteristic epidemiological features of completed
      suicide.

91.   What did Odegaard show in 1932 in relation to Norwegian
      immigrants?
      What debate did this stimulate?
      Which side did Odegaard favour for schizophrenia?

92.   List the characteristic features of institutional neurosis as
      described by Wing (1967).

93.   List the beneficial features of work as described by Jahoda and
      Rush (1980).

94.   List the characteristic epidemiological features of non-fatal
      deliberate self-harm.

95.   Write short notes on the culture-bound disorders koro, latah and
      windigo.

96.   List the characteristic features of a therapeutic community as
      originally described by Jones (1968).

97. List the clinical features of Cushing's disease.

98. List the clinical features of maple syrup urine disease. What is the enzyme deficiency, mode of inheritance and treatment of the condition?

99. List the clinical features of Huntington's chorea.

100. Write short notes on the 5 types of formal thought disorder as described by Schneider (1959).

Clinical Topics

1. Define the following sources of error in psychiatric research – Hawthorne effect, halo effect, response set and bias towards centre.

2. Define the psychiatric instrument SANS.
   List the 5 global symptoms it assesses.

3. Write short notes on the role of the clinical psychologist.

4. Define the terms mean, median, mode and range.

5. Define the terms descriptive psychopathology and dynamic psychopathology.

6. With regard to motor disorders of general behaviour, list 5 examples of non-adaptive spontaneous movements and 5 examples of non-adaptive induced movements.

7. Define the disorders of perception pareidolia and eidetic images.

8. Define the term passivity phenomena.
   List the various types.

9. List the first-rank symptoms of Schneider (1959).

10. List the characteristic features of hebephrenic, paranoid, simple and catatonic schizophrenia.

11. Write short notes on the features of a double bind as described by Bateson (1956).

12. List the distinguishing features of the conditions paranoia, paraphrenia and paranoid schizophrenia.

13. Paykel (1971) classified affective disorders by symptom clusters into 4 groups.
    Define these groups and list their characteristic features.

14. Write short notes on the 3 stages of uncomplicated bereavement reactions.

15. List the vulnerability factors for depression in Brown's study (1975) of working-class women from Inner London boroughs.

16. List and briefly define the 4 basic types of error shown by cognitive distortions in the cognitive theory of depression.

17. List the 4 characteristics of the fear in phobic disorders as described by Marks (1969).

18. Define the disorders obsessions and compulsions.

19. Define the terms hysterical dissociation and hysterical conversion.
    List the characteristic clinical features of each.

20. List the characteristic symptoms of hypochondriasis.

21. List the 8 criteria for borderline personality disorder according to DSM III.
How many criteria must be present for a diagnosis to be made?

22. List the 4 essential features of antisocial personality disorder according to DSM III.

23. List the characteristic features of schizoid personality disorder.

24. List the 3 important features of histrionic personality disorder according to DSM III.

25. Write short notes on the treatment of obesity.

26. Write short notes on the aetiology of anorexia nervosa.

27. List the clinical features of bulimia nervosa.
How does it differ from anorexia nervosa?

28. List the factors associated with a poor prognosis in anorexia nervosa.

29. List the characteristic features of the 3 groups of erectile impotence in relation to prognosis as suggested by Ansari (1976).

30. Describe briefly the 3 characteristic types of incestuous father.

31. Define the terms transvestism and transexualism.

32. List the negative aetiological factors pushing away from heterosexuality.

33. List the 7 essential elements in the alcohol dependence syndrome as described by Edwards (1977).

34. List the clinical features of delirium tremens.

35. Describe the clinical features of alcoholic hallucinosis. How do the hallucinations differ from those in the alcohol withdrawal syndrome?

36. Write short notes on the aetiology of alcohol dependence.

37. List the withdrawal effects from opiates and the clinical features of chronic opiate dependence.

38. List the withdrawal effects from barbiturates and the clinical features of barbiturate dependence.

39. Write short notes on amphetamine psychosis.

40. Write short notes on the mental effects of lysergic acid diethylamide (LSD).

41. Describe the clinical features of the Othello syndrome.

42. Write short notes on the clinical features of de Clérambault's syndrome.

43. List the clinical features of Ganser's syndrome.

44. List the clinical features of Gilles de la Tourette syndrome.

45. List the characteristic features of acute and chronic organic disorders.

46. List the characteristic features of occlusion of the anterior and middle cerebral arteries.

47. List the acute and chronic psychological effects following head injury.

48. List the clinical features of Creutzfeld – Jakob disease.

49. List the common clinical features of complex partial seizures.

50. List the ways in which hysterical seizures can be distinguished from epileptic seizures.

51. List the clinical features of narcolepsy.

52. List the clinical features of the Kleine – Levin syndrome.

53. List Post's subdivisions of elderly paranoid conditions (1966) and elderly depression (1985).

54. Write short notes on the features which distinguish depressive pseudodementia from true dementia.

55. List the characteristic features of elderly hypomania.

56. Describe the features of late paraphrenia.

57. List the 6 criteria used for determining fitness to plead in a defendant at the time of trial.

58. Define the term testamentary capacity.
List the 4 legal criteria used by doctors to decide whether or not a testator is of 'sound disposing mind'.

59. Define the terms actus reus and mens rea.
List 3 examples of crimes for which 'specific intent' is required, and 2 examples of crimes for which 'specific intent' is not required.

60. Define the term diminished responsibility.
Describe briefly how it is used as a psychiatric defence in court.

61. Describe briefly the autistic triad of infantile autism.

62. Define the term school refusal.
List the features which distinguish school-refusers from truants.

63. List the clinical features of the hyperkinetic syndrome.

64. Define the developmental delay specific reading retardation (SRR).
List the features which distinguish SRR from 'reading backwardness due to low IQ'.

65. List the characteristic features of Patau's syndrome.
    Define the genotype.

66. List the medical or surgical conditions which show increased incidence in Down's syndrome.

67. List the characteristic features of Edward's syndrome.
    Define the genotype.

68. List the clinical features of Hartnup's disease.
    What is the aetiology, mode of inheritance and treatment of the condition.

69. List the side-effects of neuroleptics.

70. List the clinical features of neuroleptic malignant syndrome (NMS).

71. List the 4 most common synthetic anticholinergic drugs used in the treatment of drug-induced parkinsonism.
    Enumerate their side-effects.

72. List the indications and side-effects of carbamazepine.

73. List the favourable features for depressive illness to respond to electroconvulsive therapy (ECT).

74. List the side-effects of ECT.

75. List the current indications for psychosurgery.
    What are the contraindications?

76. List the side-effects of psychosurgery.

77. List the 3 components of relationships, as suggested by Berne. Describe briefly the 4 stages treatment passes through in transactional group therapy, as derived from the work of Berne (1966).

78. List the therapeutic factors in small group psychotherapy, as described by Yalom (1975).

79. Define the aim of brief individual psychotherapy. Describe briefly its indications.

80 Define the term dream work in psychoanalysis. List its 5 components.

81. List the psychological and physical symptoms of premenstrual tension.

82. Define the 3 types of clinical picture observed in puerperal psychosis and indicate the predominant picture nowadays. Describe briefly the aetiology of the condition.

83. List the factors associated with puerperal depression.

84. List the particular problems of adjustment following mastectomy. Describe briefly the association between mastectomy and affective disorder.

85. Schizophrenia and depression vary in their presentation across cultures.
List the characteristic features of each illness in Africa and in India.

86. Write short notes on the culture-bound disorders amok, susto and piblokto.

87. Define the terms affect and mood according to DSM III.
List the forms mood may be expressed in, with regard to disorders of appearance and behaviour.

88. Distinguish between process schizophrenia and schizophreniform illnesses, as described by Langfeldt (1939).

89. List the 6 combinations of mixed affective states, as described by Kraepelin (1921).

90. List the factors associated with agoraphobia.

91. Define the category personality disorders, according to ICD-9 and DSM III.

92. Define the term exhibitionism.
List the aetiological factors in the condition.

93. Briefly describe Jellinek's 5 patterns of pathological drinking.

94. List the effects of cannabis.

95. Describe briefly the clinical features of 'hospital addiction syndrome'.

96. List the clinical features of Pick's disease.
Describe the pathology of the condition.

97. List the 5 diagnostic groups in psychogeriatric patients, as described by Roth (1955).

98. List the 5 types of shoplifters, as classified by Fisher (1984).

99. Write short notes on the clinical features of conduct disorders.

100. List the characteristic features of cri-du-chat syndrome.
Define the genotype.

Basic Sciences − Answers

1. Glycerophospholipids − phosphatidylcholine, phosphatidylethanolamine, phosphatidylserine, phosphatidylinositol (give any 3).

   Sphingolipids − sphingomyelins, sulphatides, gangliosides, cerebrosides (give any 3).

   Both substances are neuronal membrane lipids. Glycerophospholipids may play a role in the conduction of the nerve impulse.

   Gangliosides may be involved in calcium transport, membrane excitability and neurotransmission. Sphingomyelins are found mainly in the myelin sheath.

2. Evidence for −

   Amphetamines increase dopamine release and can produce a paranoid psychosis similar to schizophrenia. Disulfiram inhibits dopamine-beta-hydroxylase and can exacerbate schizophrenia.

   All effective neuroleptics block dopamine receptors; antipsychotic potency is related to the degree of antidopaminergic activity.

   Monoamine reuptake inhibitors can exacerbate schizophrenia.

   Post-mortem studies indicate increased dopamine levels in mesolimbic areas of schizophrenic brains.

   Evidence against −

   CSF studies fail to show increased metabolites of dopamine in schizophrenia; i.e. the levels of homovanillic acid (HVA) are reduced.

Antipsychotics may raise HVA levels.

Low-dose apomorphine, a dopamine stimulator, can lead to improvement in chronic schizophrenia.

L-DOPA can reduce the negative symptoms of schizophrenia.

3.   The substance should be present in the presynaptic nerve ending.

The substance should be released at the synapse by nerve stimulation.

The neurone should contain enzymes necessary for synthesis of the substance.

Systems should be present for inactivation of the substance.

The substance should produce the same effect as the synaptically released transmitter, when iontophoretically applied to the postsynaptic neurone (give any 4).

4.   Pyramidine bases – uracil, thymine, cytosine (give any 2).

Purine bases – guanine, adenine, xanthine (give any 2).

Processes bases are involved in – nucleic acid synthesis, neurotransmission, enzymatic reactions, energy metabolism, 'second messenger' activities, regulation of brain-blood flow (give any 4).

5.   Reserpine depletes presynaptic vesicles of monoamine stores and can result in depression.

Amphetamines cause the release of monoamines into the synaptic cleft and can result in euphoria. Monoamine oxidase inhibitors (MAOIs) and monoamine reuptake inhibitors (tricyclic antidepressants) increase the availability of monoamines to postsynaptic receptors and can elevate mood.

Post-mortem studies indicate decreased serotonin turnover in depression.

CSF and urinary studies indicate decreased levels of the breakdown products of noradrenaline and serotonin in some depressed patients.

6. Nicotinic response − stimulated by nicotine or acetylcholine, blocked by curare, always excitatory, typically quick (give any 3).

    Muscarinic response − stimulated by muscarine or acetylcholine, blocked by atropine, inhibitory or excitatory, typically slow (give any 3).

7. Serotonin − breakdown product is 5-hydroxyindolacetic acid (5-HIAA). Enzyme involved is monoamine oxidase (MAO).

    Dopamine − breakdown product is homovanillic acid (HVA). Enzymes involved are catechol-O-methyl transferase (COMT) and MAO.

    Noradrenaline − breakdown products are 3-methoxy-4-hydroxyphenylglycol (MHPG) and vanillylmandelic acid (VMA). Enzymes involved are MAO and COMT.

8. Neurotransmitters − acetylcholine, dopamine, noradrenaline, serotonin, gamma-aminobutyric acid (GABA), endorphins, prostaglandins, vasoactive intestinal peptide (VIP), substance P, neurotensin, somatostatin, histamine, cholecystokinin (CCK), glutamic acid (give any 12).

9. Intermediate substances – glucose-6-phosphate, fructose-6-phosphate, fructose-1,6-diphosphate, glyceraldehyde-3-phosphate, 1,3-diphosphoglycerate, 3-phosphoglycerate, 2-phosphoglycerate, phosphoenolpyruvate (give any 5).

10. The resting membrane potential is due to the separation of charge across the neuronal membrane. In most neurones it is about -60 mV. It is K^+ dependent.

   The action potential involves an increase in neuronal membrane permeability, with a breakdown in the ionic barrier and a resultant transient reversal of the resting membrane potential. It is Na^+-dependent.

11. Types of waves –

   Delta: less than 4 Hz
   Theta: 4 – 7.5 Hz
   Alpha: 7.5 – 13 Hz
   Beta: 13 – 40 Hz
   Mu: 7 – 11 Hz

   Delirious states are characterised by slow wave activity.

12. IPSPs – inhibitory postsynaptic potentials. These inhibit action potentials by hyperpolarising the neuronal membrane. An increase in K^+ or Cl^- permeability underlies the IPSP.

   EPSPs – excitatory postsynaptic potentials. These are depolarisations which bring the neuronal membrane closer to the threshold for action potential generation. An increase in both K^+ and Na^+ conductance underlies the EPSP.

13. Uses of EEG in psychiatry -

Detection of focal lesions e.g. frontal lobe, parietal lobe and temporal lobe lesions.

Detection of confusional states.

Diagnosis of presenile and senile dementia.

Diagnosis of epilepsy and sleep disorders.

Elimination of organic brain disease as a cause of psychotic illness.

Detection of non-organic stupor due to hysteria, schizophrenia or depression.

14. Types of synaptic contact - axo-axonic, dendro-dendritic, soma-somatic, axo-dendritic, axo-somatic.

15. Non-REM sleep EEG changes -

Stage one: low-voltage desynchronized activity. Sometimes low-voltage regular activity at 4-6 Hz.

Stage two: sleep spindles at 13-15 Hz. High-voltage K complexes.

Stage three: high-voltage, large slow, delta waves appear.

Stage four: predominantly delta waves are present.

16. Different groups -

Phenothiazines: aliphatic side chain e.g. chlorpromazine.

Phenothiazines: piperazine side chain e.g. trifluoperazine.

Phenothiazines: piperidine side chain e.g. thioridazine.

Butyrophenones e.g. haloperidol.

Thioxanthenes e.g. flupenthixol, clopenthixol.

Diphenylbutylpiperidines e.g. pimozide, fluspirilene.

Substituted benzamides e.g. sulpiride.

Other drugs e.g. rauwolfia alkaloids, tetrabenazine.

17. Biochemical actions − dopamine blocking activity, anti-adrenergic activity, anticholinergic activity, antiserotonergic activity, antihistaminergic activity.

   Largactil is so-called because of its large number of actions.

18. Clinical indications −

   Control and maintenance therapy in schizophrenia.

   Tranquillization and emergency control in behavioural disturbances.

   Short-term adjunctive treatment of severe anxiety.

   Induction of weight gain in anorexia nervosa.

   Terminal disease.

   Anti-emetic.

   Intractable hiccup.

19. Mechanism of therapeutic effects −

Decreased neurotransmitter postsynaptic receptor sensitivity.

Stimulates exit of Na^+ from cells where intracellular Na^+ is elevated (as in depression) by stimulating the Na^+/K^+ pump mechanism.

Stimulates entry of Na^+ into cells where intracellular Na^+ is reduced (as in mania).

Influences Ca^{2+} and Na^+ transfer across cell membranes including the Ca^{2+}-dependent release of neurotransmitter.

Inhibits adenyl cyclase necessary for the conversion of ATP to cyclic AMP.

Interacts with Ca^{2+} and Mg^{2+}, thereby increasing cell membrane permeability.

20. Long-term side-effects −

Nephrogenic diabetes insipidus.

Hypothyroidism.

Cardiotoxicity.

Irreversible renal damage.

Oedema.

Weight gain.

Poor short-term memory.

Tardive dyskinesia and other movement disorders.

21. Clinical indications –

    Treatment of bipolar affective disorders.

    Prophylaxis of recurrent bipolar and unipolar affective disorders.

    Treatment of mixed affective states.

    Treatment of aggressive or self-mutilating behaviour.

    Treatment of resistant depression.

22. Drugs interacting – amphetamines, common cold remedies, fenfluramine, L-DOPA, morphine, pethidine, bethanidine, guanethidine, methyldopa, tricyclic antidepressants, antihistamines, oral antidiabetic agents, tetrabenazine, reserpine (give any 10).

23. Definition – repetitive, involuntary movements of the mouth and tongue. Frequently associated with movements of the limbs and trunk. Irreversible once established.

    Possible treatments –

    Increase in neuroleptic dosage.

    Decrease in neuroleptic dosage.

    Stopping the neuroleptic completely.

    Deanol, diazepam, reserpine, tetrabenazine, barbiturate, sodium valproate (give any 7).

24.   Classification –

Tertiary amine compounds: preferentially block the reuptake of serotonin e.g. amitriptyline, imipramine, clomipramine (give any 2).

Secondary amine compounds: preferentially block the reuptake of noradrenaline and dopamine e.g. nortriptyline, desipramine, protriptyline (give any 2).

25.   Diencephalic structures – thalamus, hypothalamus, optic nerves, pituitary.

Metencephalic structures – cerebellum, pons.

Mesencephalic structures – cranial nerves III and IV, crura cerebri.

26.   Structures involved – optic nerve, optic chiasma, optic tract, pretectal nucleus, Edinger–Westpal nuclei, ciliary ganglion, eyeball, constrictor muscles of iris.

27.   Components – caudate, putamen and globus pallidus.

Principal inputs – thalamus, subthalamic nucleus, substantia nigra, cerebral cortex.

Principal outputs – thalamus, subthalamic nucleus, substantia nigra, red nucleus, reticular formation, tectum.

28.   Location – locus coeruleus in floor of 4th ventricle of pons; at least 4 groups of medullary neurones.

Projections – Locus coeruleus gives rise to the dorsal noradrenergic bundle. This innervates the thalamus, hippocampus, cerebral cortex, cerebellar cortex. Medullary neurones innervate the spinal cord, pontine reticular formation, cranial nerve nuclei, mesencephalon, pre-optic areas of hypothalamus.

29. Layers – external pyramidal layer, external granular layer, internal granular layer, multiform layer, molecular layer, ganglionic layer.

30. Structures involved – optic nerve, optic chiasma, optic tract, lateral geniculate body, visual cortex, eye field of frontal cortex, oculomotor nuclei, medial rectus muscle.

31. Components – amygdaloid nucleus, anterior nucleus of thalamus, hypothalamus, hippocampal formation; subcallosal, parahippocampal and cingulate gyri.

Principal inputs – temporal lobe, medial forebrain bundle.

Principal outputs – habenular nuclei, septal nuclei, mamillary body, tegmentum of midbrain, lateral preoptic area, reticular formation.

32. Location – ventral tegmental area, substantia nigra, arcuate nucleus of the hypothalamus.

Projections –

Ventral tegmental area neurones innervate the cerebral cortex and mesolimbic system.

Substantia nigra neurones give rise to the nigrostriatal pathway.

Arcuate nucleus neurones give rise to the tubero-infundibular system.

33. Central nuclei – arcuate, dorsomedial, paraventricular, ventromedial.

   Anterior nuclei – pre-optic, supra-optic.

   Posterior nuclei – mamillary, posterior.

34. Clinical features – depression, apathy, schizophreniform psychosis, mild cognitive impairment, anorexia, weight loss, nausea, fatigue, hypotension, hypoglycaemia, loss of body hair, impotence, vitiligo, pigmentation.

35. Hypothalamic – pituitary – thyroid axis – thyrotrophin-releasing factor (TRF) is synthesized in a number of hypothalamic areas and stored in the median eminence.

   TRF stimulates the release of thyroid-stimulating hormone (TSF) from the anterior pituitary. The neurosecretory cells of the hypothalamus control hormone release in the pituitary via the portal veins.

   The process by which iodine is trapped and used in the synthesis of thyroid hormones is under the control of TSH from the pituitary. TSH acts on a receptor site in the thyroid gland by stimulating adenyl cyclase, which converts ATP to cyclic AMP.

   Tri-iodothyronine (T_3) and thyroxine (T_4) have a negative feedback effect on the pituitary and inhibit TSH release into the portal circulation.

36. Clinical features – depression, anxiety-related symptoms, irritability, tiredness, flushing, sweating, dizziness, headache, vaginal dryness, osteoporosis, irregular periods followed by amenorrhoea.

37. Stimulatory hormones – corticotrophin-releasing factor (CRF), thyrotrophin-releasing factor (TRF), gonadotrophin-releasing hormone (GRH).

   Inhibitory hormones – melanocyte inhibitory factor (MIF), prolactin inhibitory factor (PIF); somatostatin or growth hormone inhibiting hormone (GHIH).

38. Clinical features – paroxysms of anxiety, episodic headaches, sweating, tachycardia, hypertension, weight loss.

39. Hypothalamic – pituitary – gonadal axis – gonadotrophin-releasing hormone (GRH) is synthesized in the hypothalamus.

   GRH stimulates the release of follicle-stimulating hormone (FSH) and luteinizing hormone (LH) from the anterior pituitary. The neurosecretory cells of the hypothalamus control hormone release in the pituitary via the portal veins.

   FSH and LH stimulate the development of ovarian follicles in the female; in the male they stimulate spermatogenesis and testosterone release.

   Oestrogen and progesterone have a positive feedback effect on the pituitary and stimulate FSH and LH release into the portal circulation.

   Testosterone has a negative feedback effect on the pituitary and inhibits LH release into the portal circulation.

40. Elevated hormone levels – growth hormone (GH), prolactin, cortisol.

   Reduced hormone levels – tri-iodothyronine (T_3), thyroxine (T_4), oestradiol, testosterone, follicle-stimulating hormone (FSH), luteinizing hormone (LH). (give any 6).

41. Principal genetic studies –

Family studies – these examine the factors which determine the clustering of a disease within a family. They allow the calculation of the risk of mental illness in the relatives of affected persons, on the basis of consanguinity. They do not provide a good discriminator of environmental and genetic factors in the aetiology of the illness.

Twin studies – these compare the concordance rate in monozygotic and dizygotic twins. They seek to separate environmental and genetic factors. When there is a higher concordance in monozygotic compared to dizygotic twins, there is strong evidence for genetic factors in the aetiology of the illness.

Adoption studies – these allow children who are genetically at a high risk to be studied in a family environment away from their natural parents. They seek to separate environmental and genetic factors, by reducing the influence of environmental bias in the aetiology of the illness.

42. Clinical features – fair skin, fair hair, ocular lens dislocation, iridonesis, glaucoma, malar flush, poor peripheral circulation, skeletal abnormalities, liver degeneration, epilepsy, severe mental retardation.

Enzyme deficiency – cystathionine synthetase.

Mode of inheritance – autosomal recessive.

Treatment – methionine-free diet.

43. Clinical features – gargoylism, irregular epiphyseal development, corneal clouding, cataracts, enlarged abdomen, hepatosplenomegaly, small stature, schaphocephalic skull, progressive mental and physical deterioration.

Differences – Hunter's syndrome has similar clinical features to Hurler's syndrome. However, Hunter's syndrome is usually a milder condition, there is no corneal clouding, and the rate of mental and physical deterioration is slower.

44. Clinical features – tall, thin, slightly reduced IQ, mild mental subnormality, infertile, lack of male secondary sexual characteristics, gynaecomastia, female distribution of pubic hair.

    Genotype – XXY.

45. Clinical features – fair hair, blue eyes, small stature, decreased head size, eczema, epilepsy, reduced skin pigmentation, café-au-lait spots, severe mental retardation, kyphosis, widely spaced upper incisors, brisk reflexes.

    Enzyme deficiency – phenylalanine hydroxylase.

    Mode of inheritance – autosomal recessive.

    Treatment – phenylalanine-free diet.

46. Clinical features – diarrhoea, vomiting, lethargy, failure to thrive, jaundice in neonatal period, cirrhosis, cataracts, mental retardation, early death.

    Enzyme deficiency – galactose-1-phosphate uridyl transferase.

    Treatment – galactose-free diet.

47. Clinical features – adenoma sebaceum, café-au-lait spots, shagreen patches, sclerotic brain nodules, retinal phakomata, renal tumours, variable mental retardation (mild to severe), epilepsy, schizophreniform psychosis, lung cysts.

Mode of inheritance – autosomal dominant with variable penetrance. However, 50% of cases do not have a family history and result from gene mutations.

48. Clinical features – cubitus valgus, webbed neck, gonadal dysgenesis, lack of female secondary sexual characteristics, borderline intelligence, small stature, coarction of aorta, renal malformations.

Genotype – XO.

49. Clinical features – disinhibition, facetious humour, euphoria, irritability, apathy, loss of initiative, decreased intellectual drive, loss of ethical standards, expressive dysphasia, grasp reflex, urinary incontinence, tactlessness, overtalkativeness, reduced verbal fluency, reduced fine motor control, excess in drinking and eating, excess in sexual behaviour, Gegenhalten, contralateral spastic paresis, impaired spelling, difficulty in programming and planning behaviour (give any 15).

50. Clinical features – memory failure, lability of mood, apathy, depressive or paranoid features, parkinsonism, parietal lobe dysfunction, mirror sign, logoclonia, epilepsy, relentless progress of personality and intellectual deterioration, aspects of the Klüver–Bucy syndrome.

Pathology – generalized cortical atrophy with loss of neurones, senile plaques, neurofibrillary tangles, granulovacuolar degeneration, glial proliferation, loss of dendritic branching, reduced levels of choline acetyltransferase and acetylcholinesterase.

51. Wernicke's encephalopathy – ophthalmoplegia, nystagmus, clouding of consciousness with memory disturbance, ataxia, peripheral neuropathy.

Korsakoff's psychosis – impairment of recent memory, confabulation, retrograde amnesia, disorientation, euphoria, apathy, lack of insight, ataxia, peripheral neuropathy.

52. Clinical features – euphoria, depression, impairment of recent memory, impairment of conceptual thinking, oculomotor paralysis, retrobulbar neuritis, cerebellar signs, dementia, upper motor neurone deficits, disturbance of micturition, proprioceptive loss, paraesthesia.

53. Clinical features – constructional apraxia, dressing apraxia, ideational apraxia, ideomotor apraxia, anosognosia, topographical agnosia, hemisomatognosia, autotopagnosia, sensory inattention, cortical sensory loss, astereognosis, epilepsy, aspects of Gerstmann's syndrome.

54. Clinical features – stepwise deterioration in memory, perseveration, fluctuating cognitive impairment, episodes of nocturnal confusion, depression, hypertension, headache, dizziness, tinnitus, scotomata, apraxias, agnosias, aphasia, focal neurological deficits, personality preservation until late, insight intact.

   Pathology – cerebral ischaemia and infarction, arteriosclerosis, cystic necrosis, gliosis, multiple micro-infarcts.

55. Aetiology – repeated blows to the head e.g. in boxers.

   Pathology – cerebral atrophy. Perforation of the septum pellucidum. Brainstem, hippocampus and limbic system are particularly damaged.

   Clinical features – ataxia, festinant gait, mask-like facies, 'pill-rolling' tremor, spasticity, dysarthria, epilepsy, tremor, intellectual impairment, personality deterioration, memory disturbance, persecutory ideation.

Prognosis – tends to progress insidiously.

56. Metabolic error – increased activity of delta ALA with excessive production of porphyrins, leads to porphobilinogen in the urine.

Clinical features – depression, delirium, schizophreniform psychosis, paranoid state, hypertension, abdominal pain, vomiting, constipation, bulbar palsies, peripheral neuritis, epilepsy, acute attacks precipitated by various drugs.

Mode of inheritance – autosomal dominant with variable penetrance.

57. Classical conditioning – involves the autonomic nervous system; stimulus determines the behaviour; responses are involuntary.

Operant conditioning – involves the craniospinal nervous system; behaviour determines the effect; responses are voluntary.

58. Neo-freudians – Adler, Jung, William Reich, Otto Rank, Stack-Sullivan, Horney, Fromm, Anna Freud, Melanie Klein, Bowlby (give any 6).

Post-freudians – Erikson, Winnicot, Perls-Gestalt, Rogers, Frankl, Berne, Maslow, Moreno, Assagioli, Ellis, Janov (give any 6).

59. Sensorimotor stage (0–2 years) – object constancy; object permanence; infant learns to distinguish himself from his environment.

Pre-operational stage (2–7 years) – precausal reasoning; egocentrism, animism; authoritarian morality.

Concrete operational stage (7–12 years) – child develops logical reasoning, including the laws of conservation; however, child's reasoning is still at a concrete level.

Formal operational stage (12+ years) – the child has now developed abstract reasoning.

60.   Characteristic features –

Organ inferiority and psychic compensation – personality development involves a struggle to overcome one's feelings of inferiority. All neurosis can be understood in terms of one's inferiority feelings.

Drive for superiority – the life style is the way we strive to overcome these inferiority feelings. Thus derives the importance of power and social significance in psychodynamics.

Fictive goals – the neurotic sets fictive goals and makes excuses for failing to reach them.

61.   Short-term memory – uses acoustic coding (sound); short duration (1 minute); small capacity; maintenance is by attention and rehearsal.

Long-term memory – uses semantic coding (meaning); variable duration (years); unlimited capacity; maintenance is by organization and repetition.

62.   Ego-defence mechanisms – repression, regression, projection, projective identification, displacement, denial, reaction formation, rationalization, sublimation, splitting, isolation, intellectualization, acting-out, turning on the self, distortion, identification, magic undoing (give any 12).

63.   Oral stage (0–1 years) – gratification is by oral means such as feeding and sucking; basic trust develops.

Anal stage (1-3 years) - gratification is achieved by the retention and elimination of faeces; a sense of self develops.

Phallic stage (3-5 years) - genital gratification; oedipal complex; Electra complex.

Latency period (5-12 years) - no major psychosexual development in this stage.

Genital stage (12+ years) - individual achieves full heterosexual development.

64. Stage 1 - the construction of a hierarchy of anxiety-arousing situations with the patient.

Stage 2 - the patient is taught a technique for achieving deep muscular relaxation which is incompatible with anxiety feelings e.g. Jacobsen's method.

Stage 3 - the patient is asked to visualize the first phobic item from the hierarchy whilst relaxing. This is repeated until the item no longer induces anxiety.

Stage 4 - using the same procedure, there is gradual exposure to phobic items of increasing intensity along the hierarchy, until the patient habituates and the avoidance response is extinguished.

65. Extracampine visual hallucination - a visual hallucination experienced as located outside the field of vision i.e. behind the head.

Autoscopic hallucination - the experience of seeing one's own body projected into external space, usually in front of oneself, for brief periods at a time.

Reflex hallucination - the experience of a stimulus in one sensory modality resulting in a hallucination in another sensory modality e.g. the sound of music may provoke visual hallucinations.

Complex hallucinations – the experience of a complex hallucination such as seeing faces and scenes, or hearing voices or music.

66. Loosening of associations – loss of the normal structure of thinking, muddled and illogical conversation that cannot be clarified by further enquiry. It can take several forms: knight's move or derailment, word salad or verbigeration, and talking past the point or vorbeireden.

Flight of ideas – the patient's thoughts and conversation move quickly from one topic to another, so that one train of thought is not completed before another appears. The links between these rapidly changing topics are understandable, because they occur in normal thinking i.e. rhyming, punning, clang associations and responding to distracting cues in the immediate surroundings.

Perseveration – the persistent and inappropriate repetition of the same thoughts. In response to a series of different questions the patient gives the correct answer to the first, but continues to answer subsequent questions with the answer to the first question.

67. Delusion – a false belief with the following characteristics: firmly held despite evidence to the contrary; out of keeping with the person's educational and cultural background; content often bizarre; often infused with a sense of great personal meaning.

Overvalued idea – a thought which takes precedence over others with the following characteristics: held with intense certainty, but not unshakeable conviction; understandable when the person's educational and cultural background are known; demonstrably false; has marked associated emotional investment.

68. Obsessional thoughts – repeated and intrusive words or phrases, which are usually upsetting to the patient e.g. violent, sexual and blasphemous themes.

Obsessional ruminations – repeated worrying themes of a more complex kind e.g. about the world ending.

Obsessional doubts – repeated themes expressing uncertainty about previous actions e.g. whether or not the person turned off a gas tap that might cause a fire.

Obsessional impulses – repeated urges to carry out actions that are usually dangerous, aggressive or socially embarrassing e.g. to shout obscenities in church.

Obsessional phobias – obsessional thoughts with a fearful content e.g. 'I must have AIDS'; or obsessional impulses that lead to anxiety and avoidance e.g. the impulse to stab someone with a knife and the consequent avoidance of knives.

69. Gendankenlautwerden – an auditory hallucination in which the patient experiences a voice speaking his own thoughts as he thinks them.

Écho de la pensée – an auditory hallucination in which the patient experiences a voice repeating his own thoughts immediately after he has thought them.

70. Hallucinations – perceived as being located in objective space ie. the real world; have the same 'realistic' qualities as normal perceptions; usually occur in colour; associated with a lack of insight; not subject to conscious manipulation; independent of environmental stimuli.

Pseudohallucinations – perceived as being located in subjective space i.e. within the mind; lack of solid quality of normal perceptions; usually occur in black and white; associated with the presence of insight; not subject to conscious manipulation;

independent of environmental stimuli.

71. Primary delusion – a false belief which arises fully formed as a sudden intuition, having no discernible connection with any previous interactions or experiences. Frequently preceded by a delusional mood, in which the patient feels something strange and threatening is happening, but is not sure exactly what.

Secondary delusion – a false belief which arises from some preceding morbid experience e.g. a prevailing mood, an existing delusion or a hallucination.

72. Illusion de sosies – a delusion in which a patient sees a familiar person and believes him to have been replaced by an imposter, who is an exact double of the original person.

Fregoli's illusion – a delusion in which a patient recognises a number of people as having different appearances, but believes that they are all a single persecutor in disguise.

73. Generalized anxiety disorders – 3%.

Obsessional–compulsive disorders – 0.05%.

Affective disorders – 3–4%.

Schizophrenia – 1%.

Alzheimer's disease – 5% of people over 65 years old.

74. Parametric test – assumes a normal distribution; assumes that the scores have been obtained from an interval scale of measurement i.e. a scale in which the distance between any two numbers is made up of units of known size.

Non-parametric test – uses data which are not normally distributed; the level of measurement required is ordinal i.e. the numbers need only represent the rank order of objects, on a scale from high to low.

Preference – parametric test is preferable to a non-parametric test, because the former has a greater power to detect a significant difference between two sets of scores.

75.   Reliability – the consistency with which a test obtains the result.

Types: alternate-form, inter-rater, split-half, test-retest (give any 3).

Validity – the degree to which a test measures what it is supposed to.

Types: content, construct, predictive (give any 2).

76.   Incidence – the rate of development of a disease over a period of time. Calculated by dividing the number of people who develop the disease in the time period by the total number in the population at risk.

Prevalence – the percentage of the population with the disease at a specific point in time. Calculated by dividing the number of people having the disease by the total number in the population.

77.   Case–control studies – compare groups of individuals with the disease and those without the disease. The presence of levels of relevant variables are assessed in each group.

Cohort studies – examine a group of individuals with attributes considered of interest in the origin of the disease. The group is followed up prospectively for a period of time. The development of disease within the group is noted and compared with a similar group, without the initial presence of the attributes.

Cross-sectional studies – examine the relationship between a disease and relevant variables at a particular point in time. The population sample is subdivided into groups, on the basis of the presence of suspected predisposing factors of the disease. The prevalence of the disease in each group is then compared.

78. Type I error – committed when we decide to reject the null hypothesis when it is, in fact, true.

Type II error – committed when we decide not to reject the null hypothesis when it is, in fact, false.

Inter-relationship – if we try to reduce the risk of a type I error, by lowering the probability required for significance, we automatically increase the risk of a type II error.

79. Analysis of variance (ANOVA) – a statistical method which allows one to see if the means of a number of groups differ significantly.

One-way ANOVA – used in the situation where one has k samples and wishes to see if their means differ significantly.

Two-way ANOVA – used in the situation where there are two independent variables and the levels of each are combined, so that all possible combinations are examined.

80. Target population – the whole population from whom information could be gathered.

Sample population – the subsection of a target population which is actually under study.

Random sample – selection of a sample population such that each member of the target population has an equal probability of being selected.

Stratified random sample – the target population is subdivided on the basis of specific characteristics and then randomly sampled from each stratum.

81. Axis I – major clinical psychiatric syndromes.

    Axis II – personality and specific developmental disorders.

    Axis III – physical disorders.

    Axis IV – severity of psychological stressors.

    Axis V – highest level of adaptive functioning in previous year.

82. Class 1 – dysthymic states.

    Class 2 – neurotic symptoms.

    Class 3 – integrated delusions.

    Class 4 – delusions of disintegration.

    Fould's meaning of hierarchy – the individual who fits the criteria for class 4, will also fit the criteria for classes 1, 2 and 3; insertion into a class automatically means insertion into the class beneath i.e. a high-priority condition can be accompanied by the symptoms of a low-priority condition, but only the high-priority condition need be diagnosed.

83. Categorical classification – the classification of psychiatric disorders by dividing them into categories, which are meant to represent discrete entities. The categories have been defined in terms of the symptom-patterns, course and prognosis of the different psychiatric disorders.

    Non-categorical classification – this is subdivided into dimensional and multiaxial classifications:

1. Dimensional classification – this rejects the use of separate categories. Eysenck has proposed a system of 3 dimensions: introversion – extroversion, neuroticism and psychoticism.

2. Multiaxial classification – applied to schemes of classification in which 2 or more separate sets of information (e.g. aetiology, symptoms) are coded e.g. DSM III.

84. Definition – to allocate a person to a diagnostic category is simply to add a label to deviant behaviour. The most powerful individuals within society apply labels. The least powerful individuals within society are frequently labelled.

Consequences – such labelling only serves to increase the person's difficulties e.g. terms such as schizophrenia or epilepsy attract social stigma. However, such disorders can't be made to disappear simply by ceasing to give names to them.

85. Differences –

1. In the area of affective disorders: ICD-9 classifies depression into manic depressive psychosis, psychotic depression, neurotic depression and depressive disorders not elsewhere classified. DSM III classifies depression into major affective disorders, affective personality disorders and atypical affective disorders.

2. In the area of childhood disorders: ICD-9 has 27 specific categories; DSM III has 45 specific categories.

3. Major differences exist in the areas of neurotic disorders, psychosexual disorders and organic brain syndromes.

4. Definitions of categories are far more detailed in DSM III than in ICD-9.

5.   DSM III, unlike ICD-9, gives guidance in making a differential diagnosis and points out areas of possible diagnostic error.

86.   US – UK Diagnostic Project (1972):

1.   Compared with psychiatrists in London, psychiatrists in New York diagnosed schizophrenia twice as often, and mania and depression correspondingly less often.

2.   Further investigation suggested that New York was not typical of the United States; in some other places in the United States and in Canada, diagnostic practice was closer to British practice.

International Pilot Study of Schizophrenia (1973):

1.   There was substantial agreement in diagnostic criteria in 7 of the 9 countries in the study. However, Washington and Moscow differed from the rest.

2.   In Washington – the findings confirmed the findings of the US – UK Diagnostic Project, as described above.

3.   In Moscow – psychiatrists appeared to have an unusually broad concept of schizophrenia, which reflected a particular local emphasis on the course of disorder as a diagnostic criterion.

87.   Both conditions are special diagnostic categories in France, which differ from those in Europe and the United States.

Bouffée délirante – the sudden onset of a delusional state, with trance-like feelings of short duration and good prognosis.

Délires chroniques – paranoid states subdivided into:

1. 'Focused' – with a single delusional theme.

2. 'Non-focused' – in which several areas of mental activity are affected.

88. BPRS – Brief Psychiatry Rating Scale. Consists of 19 questions which cover the spectrum of psychopathology. Ratings are made on a seven point scale (0–6). Widely used for psychiatric drug research.

PSE – present state examination. Consists of 140 items which cover a complete clinical interview. Scores are produced on 38 'syndromes'. It is most useful as a tool for the diagnosis of schizophrenia. It is less reliable in the diagnosis of neurotic disorders.

89. Class I – higher professionals and landowners.

Class II – lower professionals e.g. nurses.

Class III – skilled tradesmen.

Class IV – semi-skilled workers.

Class V – unskilled workers.

Social causation hypothesis – social conditions in lower social class areas lead to schizophrenia.

Social drift hypothesis – schizophrenia result in the individual's drift down the social scale.

90. Epidemiological features – male sex; elderly; social class I and V; urban area; loss of parent by death; socially isolated; single or widowed; physically ill; past psychiatric history; recent bereavement; premeditated setting; precipitated by guilt and hopelessness; previous suicidal attempt; incidence declining.

91. Odegaard showed an increased rate of hospital admissions for Norwegian immigrants in the United States, as compared to Norwegians at home, especially due to schizophrenia.

This stimulated debate between:

1. Social causation – environmental factors associated with migration lead to mental illness.

2. Social selection – individuals prone to or suffering from mental illness tend to migrate.

Odegaard favoured social selection for schizophrenia.

92. Characteristic features – apathy, compliance, lack of self-respect, resentment, social withdrawal, inability to care for oneself adequately, incapacity to make important decisions regarding one's future.

93. Beneficial features – imposes structure on one's day; gives the individual status; compels the individual to be active; ensures that the individual has an opportunity to socialize with others; provides goals which require the joint action of the individual with a group.

94. Epidemiological features – female sex; young; social class V; decaying inner city areas; broken home; unemployment; unstable interpersonal relationships; antisocial personality; previous criminal record for delinquent activity; major life events; impulsive setting; precipitated by situational crisis; incidence rising.

95.   Koro – occurs in Malaya and South China; an acute anxiety
      state; presents with anxiety associated with fear of the penis
      retracting into the abdomen with impending death.

      Latah – occurs in Far East and North Africa; a hysterical
      dissociative state; presents in women with echolalia, echopraxia
      and automatic obedience.

      Windigo – occurs in North American Indian tribes; a depressive
      psychosis; presents with the delusional belief that one has
      undergone mutation into a cannibalistic monster; the subject may
      attempt to act on this.

96.   Characteristic features – absence of rigid hierarchies; good
      staff – patient communication; less than 100 patients; individuals
      confronted with the results of their behaviour; rules and
      regulations arise as a result of group discussion.

97.   Clinical features – acute anxiety, paranoid features, depression,
      euphoria, hirsutism, hypertension, muscle weakness, menstrual
      irregularities, osteoporosis, obesity, purple striae, 'orange on
      stick' appearance, tendency to bruise.

98.   Clinical features – vomiting, failure to thrive, epilepsy, spasticity,
      mental retardation, rapid cerebral degeneration, paralysis, very
      early death.

      Enzyme deficiency – branched-chain ketoacid decarboxylase.

      Mode of inheritance – autosomal recessive.

      Treatment – diet low in branched-chain amino acids: leucine,
      isoleucine and valine.

99. Clinical features – insidious onset of choreo-athetoid movements; slurring of speech; ataxic gait; intention tremor; rigidity, epilepsy; apathy; depression, irritability; distractability; insidious onset of global dementia; paranoid state.

100. Derailment – a disruption of the continuity of speech by the insertion of irrelevant and inappropriate material into the stream of thought.

Drivelling – the muddling of the constituents of an idea to the extent that the meaning is totally obscured to a listener.

Desultory thinking – speech is syntactically and grammatically correct, but unrelated thoughts are inserted inappropriately into the stream of thought.

Omission – a sudden discontinuation in the stream of thought.

Substitution – the insertion of a minor thought in the place of a major thought.

Clinical Topics – Answers

1. Hawthorne effect – the researcher alters the situation by his presence.

    Halo effect – answers are chosen to 'fit' with previously chosen answers.

    Response set – subject always tends to agree or to disagree with questions.

    Bias towards centre – subject tends to choose the middle response and shun extremes.

2. Definition – scale for the assessment of negative symptoms.

    Global symptoms – affective flattening; alogia; avolition; anhedonia – associality; inattentiveness.

3. Role of clinical psychologist –

    1. Assessment of general intelligence using psychological tests – e.g. WAIS, Stanford – Binet.

    2. Assessment of personality using inventories (e.g. MMPI, EPI) and projective tests (e.g. thematic apperception test, Rorschach inkblot test).

    3. Assessment of neuropsychological status to determine the cause of cognitive deficits, using screening tests (e.g. Benton visual retention test) and batteries of tests (e.g. Luria – Nebraska battery)

    4. Assessment of aptitudes, attitudes and interests using psychological tests.

    5. Therapy – psychotherapy and behaviour therapy.

4. Mean – the sum of the sample divided by the number of observations in the sample.

    Median – the observation occurring in the middle of a sample, when the observations are arranged in rank order.

    Mode – the observation which occurs most frequently in a sample.

    Range – the difference between the largest and smallest observations in a sample.

5. Descriptive psychopathology – the objective description of abnormal states of mind. It may be seen as a scientific basis for the practice of psychiatry by defining the essential qualities of morbid mental experiences, and by understanding what the patient is experiencing. It is entirely concerned with conscious experiences and observable behaviour.

    Dynamic psychopathology – the attempt to explain the causes of abnormal states of mind in terms of psychodynamic theories of aetiology, particularly by postulating unconscious mental mechanisms.

6. Non-adaptive spontaneous movements – chorea, athetosis, orofacial dyskinesia, spasmodic torticollis, static tremor, stereotypies, tics (give any 5).

    Non-adaptive induced movements – echopraxia, echolalia, mitmachen, mitgehen, automatic obedience, forced grasping, negativism, perseveration (give any 5).

7. Pareidolia – a special type of illusion, vivid mental images occurring without conscious effort when perceiving an ill-defined stimulus e.g. the subject sees pictures in a glowing fire.

    Eidetic images – a form of pseudohallucination. Previous

perceptions are reproduced as mental images of uncanny detail and vivid intensity.

8.   Definition – the individual experiences interference with, or outside control of, his thinking, feeling, perception or behaviour. This is due to the apparent disintegration of boundaries between the self and the surrounding world.

Types – thought insertion; thought withdrawal; thought broadcasting; 'made' actions; 'made' affect; 'made' impulses; somatic passivity.

9.   First-rank symptoms –

1.   Particular forms of auditory hallucination: voices commenting on actions in the third person; voices arguing about the subject; hearing thoughts spoken aloud.

2.   Thought interference: thought insertion; thought withdrawal; thought broadcasting.

3.   Other symptoms: delusional perception; somatic hallucinations; actions or feelings experienced as made or influenced by others.

10. 1.   Hebephrenic schizophrenia – silly and childish behaviour; prominent affective symptoms and thought disorder; delusions common but unsystematized; hallucinations common but non-elaborate.

2.   Paranoid schizophrenia – prominent well-systematized persecutory or grandiose delusions or hallucinations; delusional jealousy; mood and thought processes relatively spared; patient may appear normal until his abnormal beliefs are uncovered.

3.   Simple schizophrenia – insidious development of social

withdrawal, odd behaviour and declining performance at work; absence of delusions, hallucinations and interference with thinking.

4. Catatonic schizophrenia – stupor; excitement; waxy flexibility; catalepsy; echolalia; echopraxia; automatic obedience; stereotypy; ambitendence; mannerism; mitmachen; mitgehen; negativism; perseveration.

11. Features of a double bind –

1. Occurs when an instruction is given overtly, but contradicted by a second, more covert instruction, i.e. a parent conveys two conflicting and incompatible messages to their child at the same time.

2. There is no escape from the situation in which the contradictory instructions are received.

3. The double bind leaves the child able to make only ambiguous or meaningless responses.

4. When this process persists, this was said to lead to schizophrenia.

12. Paranoia – delusions present; hallucinations absent; personality intact.

Paraphrenia – delusions present; hallucinations present; personality intact.

Paranoid schizophrenia – delusions present; hallucinations present; personality deterioration.

13. Younger depressives with personality disorder – fluctuating mood; disturbed relationships; young.

Hostile depressives – hostile; young.

Anxious depressives – anxiety and motor agitation; moderate depression; middle age.

Psychotic depressives – prominent perceptual, biological or behavioural symptoms.

14. First stage – 'stunned' phase. Characterized by a lack of emotional reaction (i.e. blunted emotions) and a feeling of unreality. Lasts from a few hours to two weeks.

    Second stage – mourning phase. Characterized by sadness, weeping, anorexia, disturbed sleeping pattern, motor restlessness, irritability, impaired concentration and difficulty in remembering. There is also a preoccupation with the deceased, in the form of transient hallucinatory episodes and guilt or denial.

    Third stage – acceptance and readjustment phase. The symptoms of the mourning phase subside gradually and the person accepts the new situation. Complete readjustment occurs several weeks after the onset of the mourning phase.

15. Vulnerability factors –

    Three or more children under 15 years of age at home.

    Not working outside the home.

    Lack of a supportive relationship with husband.

    Loss of mother by death or separation before the age of 11.

    An excess of threatening life events or major difficulties prior to the onset of depression.

16. Arbitrary inference – drawing a conclusion when there is no evidence for it and even some against it.

Selective abstraction – focusing on a detail and ignoring more important features of a situation.

Over-generalization – drawing a general conclusion on the basis of a single incident.

Minimization and magnification – performance is underestimated and errors are overestimated.

17. Characteristics of the fear –

It is out of proportion to the demands of the feared situation.

It leads to an avoidance of the feared situation.

It cannot be explained or reasoned away.

It is beyond voluntary control.

18. Obsessions – recurrent, persistent thoughts, impulses, or images that the patient regards as absurd and alien (ego-alien), while recognizing them as the product of his own mind (ego-syntonic). Attempts are made (at least early on) to resist or ignore them. Frequently the obsessions are of an aggressive or sexual nature.

Compulsions – the motor component of an obsessional thought.

19. Hysterical dissociation – an apparent dissociation between different mental activities. The major dissociative reactions are psychogenic amnesia, psychogenic fugue, somnabulism and multiple personality.

Hysterical conversion – the term stems from Freud's theory that mental energy can be converted into certain physical symptoms.

'Classic' conversion symptoms are paralysis, fits, blindness, deafness, aphonia, anaesthesia, abdominal pain and disorders of gait.

20.   Characteristic symptoms –

1.   Pain – common sites are the right iliac fossa, lower lumbar region and the head.

2.   Worries about bladder function.

3.   Complaints about appearance – especially the shape of the breasts, nose or ears.

4.   Complaints about sweating or body odour.

5.   Cardiovascular symptoms – dyspnoea, left-sided chest pain, palpitations, worries about blood pressure.

6.   Gastrointestinal symptoms – acid regurgitation, biliousness, nausea, bad taste in mouth, abdominal pain, flatulence, dysphagia.

21.   Criteria – unstable relationships, undue anger, variable moods, chronic boredom, doubts about personal identity, intolerance of being left alone, self-injury, impulsive behaviour which is damaging to the person.

5 criteria must be present.

22.   Essential features – impulsive actions, lack of guilt, failure to make loving relationships, failure to learn from adverse experiences.

23.   Characteristic features – introspective; prone to engage in an inner world of fantasy rather than take action; lack of emotional warmth and rapport; self-sufficient and detached; aloof and humourless; incapable of expressing tenderness or affection; shy; often eccentric; insensitive; ill at ease in company.

24.   Important features – self-dramatization; a self-centred approach to personal relationships; a craving for excitement and novelty.

25.   Mildly obese: advice about diet.

Moderately obese:

1.   Careful calorie-controlled diet.

2.   Psychotherapy – group psychotherapy; marital therapy to alter family patterns; inpatient supervision in therapeutic milieu.

3.   Behaviour therapy – makes use of positive rewards for weight loss or for behaviour that reduces the likelihood of eating e.g. eating exceptionally slowly.

4.   Pharmacotherapy – appetite-suppressing drugs e.g. fenfluramine, phentermine.

Grossly obese:

1.   Jaw-wiring.

2.   By-pass operations – truncal vagotomy; gastric partition or bypass; jejuno-ileal bypass.

26.   Aetiology

1.   Genetic – 6–10% of female siblings of patients with established anorexia nervosa suffer with the condition.

2.   Hypothalamic dysfunction – with abnormal control of food intake and reduced sex hormones, which show delayed return on recovery of normal weight.

3.   Social factors – high prevalence in upper and middle social classes; high prevalence in occupational groups particularly concerned with weight e.g. ballet students.

4.   Individual psychological causes –

   a.   Disturbance of body image – of which the 3 predisposing factors are – dietary problems in early life; parents who are preoccupied with food; family relationships that leave the child without a sense of identity.

   b.   Analytical model – regression to childhood; fixation at oral (pregenital) level of psychosexual development; escape from the emotional problems of adolescence.

5.   Causes within the family –

   a.   A specific pattern of relationships could be identified – consisting of enmeshment, overprotectiveness, rigidity and lack of conflict resolution.

   b.   Development of anorexia nervosa in patient serves to prevent dissention within the family.

27. Clinical features – binge eating often of high calorie foods and covertly; bouts of dieting, self-induced vomiting or purgative abuse in an attempt to compensate for binge eating; complications of repeated vomiting: cardiac arrythmias, renal damage, urinary infections, pitted teeth, epileptic fits, tetany, weakness.

Differences from anorexia nervosa – patients are usually eager for help; menstrual abnormalities occur in less than half the patients; bodyweight usually within normal limits.

28. Poor prognostic factors – long illness; late age of onset; bulimia; vomiting or purging; anxiety when eating in presence of others; great weight loss; poor childhood social adjustment; poor parental relationships; male sex.

29. Group 1 – good prognosis with treatment, unlikely to relapse; younger age group (average 30); acute onset with precipitant present; often unmarried; short duration.

Group 2 – good prognosis with treatment, but likely to relapse; older age group (average 45); insidious onset with chronic relationship problems; often reduced sexual response in partner.

Group 3 – poor prognosis, unlikely to respond to treatment; older age group (average 45); insidious onset with no discernible precipitant present; often history of low sex drive.

30. Paedophilic type – attracted to his daughters due to paedophilia.

Promiscuous type – incestuous activity is part of general hedonism; ignores sexual taboos.

Endogamic type – confines all his social and sexual activities to his family; often a yearning for a sexually inaccessible person.

31. Transvestism – disorder of general role behaviour. Repeated dressing in clothes of the opposite sex. Varies from occasional wearing of a few articles of clothing to complete cross-dressing.

    Transexualism – disorder of core gender identity. The transexualist is convinced he is of the sex opposite to that indicated by his normal external genitalia. He feels estranged from his body, has an overpowering desire to live as a member of the opposite sex, and looks to alter his external genitalia and bodily appearance to conform to those of the opposite sex.

32. Negative aetiological factors – failure of heterosexual relationships; lack of confidence in masculinity and potency; incestuous feelings towards mother leading to guilt; learned inhibition within the family.

33. Essential elements – subjective awareness of compulsion to drink; stereotyped pattern of drinking; increased tolerance to alcohol; primacy of drinking over other activities; repeated withdrawal symptoms; relief drinking; reinstatement after abstinence.

34. Clinical features – clouding of consciousness; disorientation in time and place; impairment of recent memory; illusions; hallucinations; delusions; agitation and restlessness; fearful affect; prolonged insomnia; tremulous hands; truncal ataxia; autonomic overactivity.

35. Clinical features – auditory hallucinations occurring alone in clear consciousness. Voices usually utter insults or threats; may be followed by secondary delusional interpretation. The patient is usually distressed by these experiences, appearing anxious and restless.

    Differences – the auditory hallucinations in simple withdrawal states and delirium tremens are fleeting and disorganized. The auditory hallucinations experienced in alcoholic hallucinosis are persistent and organized.

36.　1.　Genetic factors – twin studies show higher concordance rates in MZ than DZ twins. An adoption study by Goodwin (1973) showed significantly higher levels of alcoholism in individuals whose biological parents were known alcoholics and who were adopted in childhood, than in a matched control group.

　　2.　Biochemical factors – abnormalities in alcohol dehydrogenase or in neurotransmitter mechanisms.

　　3.　Learning factors – children tend to follow their parents' drinking patterns.

　　4.　Personality factors – alcohol dependence associated with chronic anxiety, self-indulgent tendencies and a pervading sense of inferiority.

　　5.　Psychiatric illness – alcohol dependence occurs in patients with anxiety states (including social phobias), affective disorders, schizophrenia and organic brain disease.

　　6.　Alcohol consumption in society – rate of alcohol dependence is related to the general level of alcohol consumption in society.

37.　Withdrawal effects – pilo-erection; shivering; abdominal cramps; diarrhoea; lacrimation; rhinorrhoea; dilated pupils; tachycardia; yawning; intense craving for drug; agitation; restlessness.

Chronic opiate dependence – constipation; constricted pupils; chronic malaise; weakness; impotence; tremors.

38.   Withdrawal effects – clouding of consciousness; disorientation; hallucinations; major seizures; anxiety and restlessness; pyrexia and tremulousness; insomnia and hypotension; nausea; vomiting; anorexia; twitching.

Barbiturate dependence – slurred speech; incoherence; dullness; drowsiness; nystagmus; depression.

39.   Amphetamine psychosis:

1.   Excessive or chronic use of amphetamines, whether taken by mouth or intravenously, induces a paranoid psychosis indistinguishable from acute paranoid schizophrenia.

2.   Features – hostile and dangerously aggressive behaviour; prominent persecutory delusions; auditory, visual and tactile hallucinations; clear consciousness.

3.   The condition usually subsides on discontinuing the drug over about a week. However, a few cases continue for months.

4.   It is uncertain whether amphetamine psychosis is a case of schizophrenia provoked by amphetamines, or a true drug-induced psychosis.

40.   Mental effects of LSD:

1.   Develop during the 2 hours after LSD consumption; usually last from 8 to 14 hours.

2.   Unpredictable and extremely dangerous behaviour; the user sometimes injuring or killing himself through behaving as if he were invulnerable.

3.   Mood – acute anxiety, distress or exhilaration.

4.   Distortions or intensifications of sensory perception –

a.   Synaesthesia – confusion between sensory modalities e.g. movements are experienced as if heard.

b.   Distortion of the body image – the person sometimes feels that he is outside his own body. These experiences may lead to panic with fears of insanity.

41.   Clinical features –

1.   Essential feature – a delusional belief that the marital partner is being unfaithful.

2.   This may be accompanied by other delusions – that the spouse is trying to poison the patient, plotting against him, infecting him with venereal diseaese, or taking away his sexual capacities.

3.   Behaviour – intensive seeking for evidence of partner's infidelity e.g. by examining sexual organs, underwear or bed-linen for signs of sexual secretions. The patient has the desire to extract a confession from the spouse. This may lead to severe aggression and murder.

4.   Mood – mixture of anger, apprehension, irritability and misery.

42.   Clinical features –

1.   Essential feature – a delusional belief that another person (the object), often of unattainably higher social status, loves the patient (the subject) intensely.

2.   The subject is usually a single woman.

3.   The subject believes she has been specially chosen by the object, and that it was not she who made the initial advances.

4. The subject is convinced that the object cannot be happy or a complete person without her.

5. The subject believes that the object is unable to reveal his love to her.

6. The subject may be importunate and disrupt the object's life.

7. After rejection by the object, the subject's feelings may turn to hatred.

43. Clinical features – the giving of approximate answers i.e. answers to simple questions that are plainly wrong but strongly suggest that the correct answer is known; apparent clouding of consciousness; hysterical dissociative symptoms (e.g. psychogenic amnesia); hysterical conversion symptoms (e.g. ataxia); pseudohallucinations.

44. Clinical features – multiple tics; vocaltics (grunting, snarling); echolalia; echopraxia; coprolalia (obscene utterances); stereotyped movements (dancing, jumping); learning difficulties; emotional disturbances; overactivity.

45. Acute organic disorder – acute onset; fluctuating course; perceptual abnormalities; impaired consciousness.

Chronic organic disorders – insidious onset; steady progressive course; global impairment of cerebral functions; clear consciousness.

46. Anterior cerebral artery – contralateral lower limb paresis and sensory deficits; clouding of consciousness.

Middle cerebral artery – contralateral hemiplegia, hemianaesthesia and hemianopia; clouding of consciousness;

motor and sensory aphasia if dominant cerebral hemisphere affected.

47. Acute psychological effects – impaired consciousness; retrograde amnesia (loss of memory for events prior to injury); post-traumatic or anterograde amnesia (inability to memorize ongoing events); acute post-traumatic psychosis.

   Chronic psychological effects – personality changes; chronic neurosis; affective or schizophreniform psychoses; lasting cognitive impairment.

48. Clinical features – personality change; intellectual deterioration; spasticity; cerebellar ataxia; dysphagia; dysarthria; seizures; myoclonic jerks; parietal signs; psychotic features; memory loss; extrapyramidal features (rigidity, tremor, mask-like facies).

49. Clinical features –

   1. Aura – 'epigastric aura' i.e. a sensation of churning felt in the stomach and spreading towards the neck.

   2. Affective – anxiety, fear.

   3. Thoughts – delusions.

   4. Perceptual – gustatory or olfactory hallucinations; depersonalization or derealization; déjà vu.

   5. Cognitive – fugues in which wandering is associated with narrowing of consciousness; automatisms in which the maintenance of posture and the performance of simple or complex actions without awareness, is associated with clouding of consciousness.

   6. First rank symptoms of schizophrenia.

50. Distinguishing features – there is no urinary incontinence, injury or cyanosis; the tongue is not bitten; the pattern of movements does not show a regular and stereotyped form of seizure; the patient may seem inaccessible but does not become unconscious; the patient screams during an attack rather than at the onset; the seizure is caused by emotional disturbance; EEG findings are normal.

51. Clinical features –

   1. Day-time attacks of irresistible sleep.

   2. Cataplexy – a sudden reduction in muscle tone; the patient may fall to the ground.

   3. Sleep paralysis – a marked reduction in muscle tone, usually on waking.

   4. Hypnagogic hallucinations – usually auditory.

52. Clinical features – episodes of pathological overeating and hypersomnia; irritability on waking and occasionally aggressiveness; hypersexuality; mood disturbances (e.g. depression); hallucinations; disorientation.

53. Elderly paranoid conditions – schizophrenia with first-rank symptoms; schizophrenia with paranoid symptoms; paranoid hallucinosis.

   Elderly depression – agitated depression; masked depression; organic depression; depressive pseudodementia; senile melancholia.

54. Distinguishing features –

1. Conspicuous subjective difficulty in concentration and remembering – but careful clinical testing shows there is no defect of memory function.

2. Psychological symptoms precede the apparent intellectual defects – hence it is important to interview other informants to determine the precise mode of onset.

3. Relatively acute onset.

4. Absence of focal signs.

5. Abreaction or sleep deprivation may clarify the diagnosis.

55. Characteristic features –

1. Clinical picture nearly always combines manic and depressive symptoms.

2. May present as 'confusion' and possibly delirium.

3. Speech – garrulous and anecdotal.

4. Mood – claim to be happy; however appear irritable, tense and miserable, often without any infectious gaiety ('miserable mania').

5. Thought content – persecutory or sexual preoccupations or delusions.

6. Thought form – little flight of ideas.

56. Features –

1. Schizophrenia-like disorders of volition, affect and thought.

2. Conspicuous hallucinations.

3. Relatively good preservation of personality, memory and intellect.

4. Chronic course.

5. Regarded as the mode of manifestation of schizophrenia in old age.

6. Less severe cases – regarded as eccentricity and not brought to medical attention.

57. Fitness to plead involves being able to –

1. Understand the nature of the charge.

2. Understand the significance of the plea i.e. understand the difference between pleading guilty and not guilty.

3. Examine a witness.

4. Challenge a juror.

5. Instruct counsel.

6. Follow the evidence presented in court.

58. Definition – testamentary capacity refers to the capacity of a person to make a valid will.

Legal criteria –

1. Whether the testator knows the nature and extent of his or her property, though not in detail.

2. Whether the testator knows the names of persons having a claim on his or her property, and can assess the relative

strengths of their claims.

3. Whether the testator can express himself or herself clearly and without ambiguity i.e. whether the testator is free from an abnormal state of mind that might distort judgements of feelings relevant to making the will.

4. Whether the testator understands what a will is, and what its consequences are.

59. Definitions – before a person can be convicted of a crime, the prosecution must prove:

1. Actus reus – that the person carried out an unlawful act.

2. Mens rea – that the person had specific guilty intent at the time i.e. a certain guilty state of mind.

Crimes for which 'specific intent' is required – murder, assault with intent to cause grevious bodily harm, rape, arson (give any 3).

Crimes for which 'specific intent' is not required – manslaughter, assault occasioning actual bodily harm, indecent assault, some types of traffic offences (give any 2).

60. Definition – at the material time the accused was suffering from such 'abnormality of mind' as substantially to impair his mental responsibility for his acts. 'Abnormality of mind' is a state of mind so different from that of ordinary human beings, that the reasonable person would term it abnormal.

Use as a psychiatric defence –

1. If a person is charged with murder – on the grounds of diminished responsibility, he may plead that he is not guilty of murder but guilty of manslaughter.

2. If the plea is acceptable to the prosecution and to the judge – there is no trial and a sentence for manslaughter is passed.

3. If the plea is not acceptable to the prosecution or to the judge – a trial is held.

   a. If the accused is convicted of manslaughter – the judge may pass whatever sentence he deems appropriate.

   b. If the accused is convicted of murder – there is a statutory sentence of life imprisonment.

61. Autistic triad –

1. Autistic aloneness – the inability to make warm emotional relationships with people. A characteristic sign is gaze avoidance i.e. the absence of eye to eye contact.

2. Obsessive desire for sameness – describes stereotyped behaviour together with evidence of distress, if there is any change in the environment.
   Autistic children are often fascinated by spinning toys.

3. Speech and language disorder – speech may develop late or never appear.
   This lack of speech is a manifestation of a severe cognitive defect, which affects non-verbal communication as well.

62. Definition – persistent refusal or reluctance to go to school, in order to stay with major attachment figure at home.

Distinguishing features – compared with the truants, the school-refusers:

1. Come from more neurotic families.

2. Are more depressed.

3. Have better records of school work.

4. Have better records of behaviour at school.

5. Are overprotected.

6. Are passive.

7. Stay at home.

63. Clinical features –

Extreme restlessness.

Prolonged and sustained motor overactivity.

Poor concentration and distractability.

Learning difficulties – due in part to impaired attention.

Minor forms of antisocial behaviour – especially aggression and disobedience.

Fluctuating mood – often one of depression.

Temper tantrums.

64. Definition – applies to children whose reading ability falls significantly below the average for their age, schooling and IQ; a reading age for 10-year-olds of 28 months or more below the level expected from the child's age and IQ.

Distinguishing features – compared to children whose reading backwardness is due to low IQ, children with SRR:

1. Are more often boys.

2.   Are more likely to have minor neurological abnormalities.

3.   Are less likely to come from socially disadvantaged homes.

4.   Have impairment of reading, writing and spelling, but no impairment of development in other areas.

65.   Characteristic features – cleft lip and cleft palate, small eyes and cataracts, microcephaly, congenital heart disease, polydactyly, myoclonic spasms, deafness, severe mental retardation.

Genotype – trisomy 13.

66.   Increased incidence of – umbilical hernia, blepharitis, cataracts, congenital heart disease, gastrointestinal atresia, Hirschsprung's disease, acute leukaemia, lymphocytic thyroiditis, Alzheimer's dementia, epilepsy, respiratory infections.

67.   Characteristic features – webbing of the neck, shield-shaped chest, micrognathia, wide skull in A – P diameter, short fingers, short toes, congenital heart disease, severe mental retardation.

Genotype – trisomy 18.

68.   Clinical features – depression, psychosis, confusion, mental retardation, nystagmus, ataxia, pyramidal signs, pellagra, photosensitive skin.

Aetiology – deficiency of transport of amino acids across the gut and the kidney tubules. This leads particularly to low tryptophan absorption from the gut and resorption from the kidney tubules, and abnormal amino acids in the urine.

Mode of inheritance – autosomal recessive.

Treatment – high protein diet and nicotinamide.

69. Side-effects -

Extrapyramidal side-effects - acute dystonic reactions, akathisia, pseudoparkinsonism, tardive dyskinesia.

Anticholinergic side-effects - dry mouth, blurred vision, constipation, urinary retention, tachycardia, impotence.

Anti-adrenergic side-effects - postural hypotension, failure of ejaculation.

Elevated prolactin levels - galactorrhoea in women, gynaecomastia in men.

Cardiac anomalies.

Cholestatic jaundice.

Bone marrow suppression - leucopenia.

Retinitis pigmentosa - particularly induced by thioridazine.

Epilepsy.

Weight gain.

Impaired temperature regulation - hypothermia or hyperpyrexia.

Skin photosensitivity and pigmentation.

70. Clinical features - hyperthermia, fluctuating level of consciousness, muscular rigidity, akinesia, pallor, sweating, tachycardia, labile blood pressure, increased respiration, urinary incontinence.

71. Most commonly used drugs - procyclidine, orphenadrine, benzhexol, benztropine.

Side-effects –

1. Anticholinergic side-effects – dry mouth, blurred vision, constipation, retention in prostatic hypertrophy, tachycardia, exacerbation of glaucoma.

2. Exacerbation of tardive dyskinesia.

3. Mental confusion, excitement and psychiatric disturbances – with high doses in susceptible patients; these side-effects may necessitate discontinuation of treatment.

4. Acute organic syndromes – particularly in the elderly.

5. Sweating, dizziness.

6. Hypersensitivity, nervousness.

7. Gastrointestinal disturbances.

8. Hepatic enzyme induction – leading to decreased serum levels of phenothiazine.

72. Indications –

1. All forms of epilepsy – except absence seizures.

2. Trigeminal neuralgia.

3. Prophylaxis of recurrent bipolar and unipolar affective disorders.

4. Treatment of resistant depression.

5. Behavioural disorders secondary to limbic epileptic instability.

Side-effects –

1. Dizziness and drowsiness.

2. Generalized erythematous rash.

3. Visual disturbances.

4. Gastrointestinal disturbances.

5. Leucopenia and other blood disorders.

73. Favourable features – early morning wakening, weight loss, appetite loss, psychomotor retardation, self-reproach, paranoid features, somatic delusions, loss of insight, sudden onset, duration of illness less than 1 year, positive family history, 'pyknic' build, obsessional personality.

74. Side-effects – headache, anxiety, retrograde amnesia, anterograde amnesia, nausea, vertigo, confusion, muscle pain, damage to teeth, lips or tongue, electrical burns, crush fractures of vertebrae, dislocation, fat embolism, mania in bipolar subjects.

75. Indications – persistent depression, persistent anxiety states, persistent obsessional – compulsive disorders.

    Contraindications – diffuse brain damage, cerebrovascular disease, alcoholism, drug addiction, psychopathic disorder, 'poor impulse control'.

76. Side-effects – apathy, excessive weight gain, disinhibition, emotional lability, incontinence, epilepsy.

77.   Three components –

    1.   Residues of childhood behaviour.

    2.   Remains of earlier relationships with parents.

    3.   Adult level of interaction.

Four stages –

    1.   Structural analysis – encourages each member of the group to recognise the 3 components of relationships in himself.

    2.   Transactional analysis – deals with the ways in which group members relate to one another.

    3.   Game analysis – examines transactions between several people.

    4.   Script analysis – examines a 'script' i.e. a consistent pattern of interaction laid down in childhood and persisting into adult life.

78.   Therapeutic factors – cohesiveness, interpersonal learning, universality, altruism, modelling, catharsis, existential awareness, instillation of hope, guidance, insight, development of socializing techniques, corrective recapitulation of primary family group.

79.   Aim – to produce limited but definite changes in the patient's ways of dealing with situations that cause him distress.

Indications –

    1.   Mainly helpful for patients who have difficulties in personal relationships, but are free from serious disorder of personality.

2. Especially suitable for patients who have problems in relationships leading to unhappiness and anguish, in the absence of a specific neurotic syndrome.

80. Definition – the process which turns the hidden 'latent content of the dream' into the reported 'manifest content of the dream'.

Components – condensation, displacement, dramatization, symbolization, secondary elaboration.

81. Psychological symptoms – anxiety, depression, irritability, forgetfulness, tiredness.

Physical symptoms – breast tenderness, feeling bloated, headache, backache, weight gain, abdominal discomfort.

82. Clinical picture – affective, schizophrenic and acute organic.

Nowadays – affective picture predominates.

Aetiology –

1. Genetic factors – a family history of major psychiatric illness predisposes to puerperal psychosis. Thus, genetic factors appear to play a part in the aetiology of the illness.

2. Biochemical factors – the sudden decrease in oestrogen and progesterone after childbirth affects tryptophan metabolism. Thus, biochemical factors may precipitate puerperal psychosis in predisposed women.

3. Psychological factors – death of the baby may be a clear precipitant.

4. Psychodynamic factors –

    a. The patient's relationship with her own mother.

b.　　The patient's relationship with her husband and his personality.

c.　　The patient's feelings about the responsibility of motherhood, and her reaction to this assertion of her female role.

83.　Factors – severe postpartum 'blues', past history of psychiatric illness, increased age, a tendency to more neurotic and less extroverted personalities, poor marital relationship and absence of social support, physical problems in the pregnancy and perinatal period, childhood separation from father, relationship problems with mother and father-in-law, recent stressful life events, mixed feelings about the baby.

84.　Problems – low self-esteem, embarrassment about disfigurement, sexual problems, marital problems.

Association –

1.　　About 25% of patients undergoing mastectomy develop an affective disorder within 18 months.

2.　　Affective symptoms are particularly common:

a.　　After a recurrence.

b.　　During chemotherapy and radiotherapy.

85.　Schizophrenia –

1.　　In Africa – excitement, unsystematized delusions (often persecutory), transient hallucinations, confusion.

2.　　In India – catatonic symptoms.

Depression –

1. In Africa – paranoia, hypochondriasis.

2. In India – somatic complaints (stomach pains; sexual dysfunction in men), agitation, hypochondriasis.

86. Amok –

1. Occurs in South East Asia.

2. A hysterical dissociative state or a depressive state.

3. Presents with a depressive withdrawal followed by an outburst of aggressive and frequently homicidal behaviour.

4. Usually ends with the individual killing himself or being killed.

Susto –

1. Occurs in Central and South America.

2. An acute anxiety state.

3. Presents with anxiety and fear attributed to the loss of the soul – possibly due to individual's inability to fulfil his or her expected social role.

Piblokto –

1. Occurs in Eskimo women.

2. A hysterical dissociative state.

3. Results in suicidal or homicidal behaviour.

87.   Affect – short-term disorder of emotion.

Mood – sustained disorder of emotion.

Forms –

1.   Appearance – facial expression, posture.

2.   Manner – response to others.

3.   Motility – degree and form of movements.

88.   Process schizophrenia – poor prognosis, insidious onset, lack of initiative, emotional blunting, primary delusions, paranoid symptoms, chronic hallucinations, derealization, absence of organic disease.

Schizophreniform illnesses – good prognosis, acute onset, presence of a precipitating factor, hysterical symptoms, affective symptoms prominent, clouding of consciousness.

89.   6 combinations – manic stupor, anxious mania, unproductive mania, inhibited mania, excited/agitated depression, depression with flight of ideas.

90.   Factors –

1.   Social or emotional problems e.g. worry about a sick child.

2.   Stable families.

3.   Often precipitated by major life events.

4.   Anxious, dependent and passive premorbid personalities.

5.   Concurrent physical illness.

6. Recent childbirth.

7. History of enuresis and childhood fears.

8. Higher incidence of sexual problems in female group, compared to control population.

9. Similar to general population in terms of social class and education.

91. Definition –

Deeply ingrained, maladaptive patterns of behaviour.

Recognizable in adolescence or earlier.

Continuing throughout most of adult life.

Either the patient or others have to suffer.

There is an adverse effect on the individual or society.

92. Definition – the repeated exposing of the genitals by an adult male in the presence of an unwilling female, for the purposes of achieving sexual excitement but not as a prelude to sexual intercourse.

Aetiological factors –

1. Failure to resolve oedipal conflict.

2. General inhibition of social relationships.

3. Enjoyment of risk taking.

4. Poor sexual performance.

5. Unduly close ambivalent relationship with mother.

6.   Poor distant relationship with ineffectual father.

7.   Personality factors – lack of assertion, passive, immature, obsessional.

8.   Dissociative behaviour in response to stress or depression.

9.   Witness response may reinforce behaviour.

93.   5 patterns –

1.   Alpha – purely psychological dependence. No loss of control drinking.

2.   Beta – physical complications. No physical dependence.

3.   Gamma – loss of control drinking with withdrawal symptoms. Ability to abstain.

4.   Delta – inability to abstain with withdrawal symptoms. Comparatively little social disruption.

5.   Epsilon – bout drinking.

94.   Effects –

1.   Exaggerates the pre-existing mood – whether euphoria, depression or anxiety.

2.   Distortion of time and space.

3.   Increased enjoyment of aesthetic experiences.

4.   Intensification of visual perception and visual hallucinations.

5.   Dry mouth.

6. Coughing.

7. Increased appetite.

8. Decreased body temperature.

9. Reddening of the eyes.

10. Irritation of the respiratory tract.

95. Clinical features –

1. Patient repeatedly presents himself at hospitals with dramatic symptoms suggesting serious acute physical illness.

2. These symptoms seem to require urgent surgical treatment or the administration of powerful analgesics.

3. Commonest symptoms – acute abdominal or loin pain, haemoptysis, haematemesis.

4. Patient shows extensive pathological lying and lack of personal rapport.

5. Variants of the syndrome present with false bereavements or psychiatric symptoms.

96. Clinical features – frontal lobe syndrome, personality deterioration, nominal aphasia, perseveration, amnesia, generalized hyperalgesia.

Pathology –

1. Atrophy confined to frontal and temporal lobes.

2. Knife blade atrophy – due to neuronal loss.

3.   Pick's cells – swollen cells with argentophile inclusion bodies.

4.   Fibrous gliosis.

97.   Diagnostic groups – senile psychosis, arteriosclerotic psychosis, affective psychosis, late paraphrenia, acute confusion.

98.   Types – professional shoplifters, young shoplifters, reactive shoplifters, shoplifters with severe psychiatric disorders, shoplifters with abnormal learned behaviour.

99.   Clinical features –

1.   Severe and persistent antisocial behaviour which is more serious than ordinary childish mischief and attracts social disapproval – stealing, lying, disobedience, truancy, verbal or physical aggression, setting fire, alcohol and drug abuse, reckless behaviour, poor school work, delinquency, masturbation and sexual curiosity, promiscuity, vandalism.

2.   The antisocial behaviour in conduct disorders must be associated with disturbances of personal functioning or subjective happiness, to distinguish it from law-breaking behaviour i.e. delinquency.

100.   Characteristic features – cat-like cry, congenital heart disease, small hands, small feet, microcephaly, epilepsy, facial abnormalities, spasticity, severe mental retardation, compatible with adult life.

Genotype – deletion of the short arm of chromosome 5.